THE 31-DAY GUIDE TO CAREGIVING

Mary Banks

Order this book online at www.trafford.com
or email orders@trafford.com

Most Trafford titles are also available at major online book retailers.

Print information available on the last page.

ISBN: 978-1-6987-1757-9 (sc)
ISBN: 978-1-6987-1758-6 (e)

Trafford rev. 09/03/2024

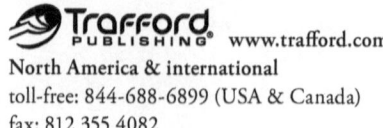

www.trafford.com
North America & international
toll-free: 844-688-6899 (USA & Canada)
fax: 812 355 4082

PRAYER IS VERY IMPORTANT!

PRAY EVERYDAY FOR PATIENCE; BE GRATEFUL THAT THE LORD TRUST YOU WITH SUCH A TASK. IT IS A PRIVILEGE TO BE ABLE TO CARE AND SUPPORT ANOTHER HUMAN BEING. LOVE MUST BE ATTACHED TO YOUR WORK.

EACH DAY YOUR ROUTINE MAY BE THE SAME; HOWEVER, EACH DAY IS SLIGHTLY DIFFERENT. THE MOOD OF YOUR CLIENT CHANGES BY THE MINUTE. IT IS YOUR JOB TO ENCOURAGE THEM TO GET OUT OF THE BED, SHOWER, MOISTERIZE, BRUSH THEIR TEETH, COMB HAIR, DRESS AND PUT SHOES ON THEIR FEET.

EVEN BEDRIDDEN PATIENTS
MUST BE CLEAN DAILY.

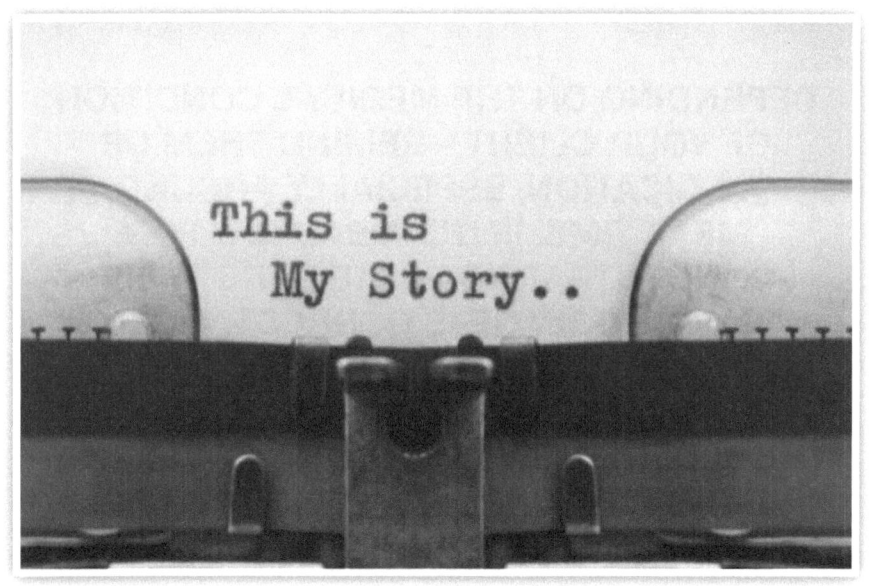

DEPENDING ON THE MEDICAL CONDITION OF YOUR CLIENT – REMIND THEM OF MEDICATION, ESPECIALLY AROUND MEAL TIME. IF IT'S A BAD DAY FOR CONCENTRATING, MAKE SURE THEIR MEDICINE DOSAGE IS CORRECT AND YOU MAY HAVE TO SELECT A BETTER DAY FOR THEM TO MAKE BUSINESS CALLS. MANY OF THE ELDERLY HAVE DEMENTIA AT VARIOUS DEGREES AS WELL AS OTHER ISSUES.

MAKE SURE THAT THE CLIENT CONFIRMS ALL DOCTOR'S APPOINTMENTS, ESPECIALLY IF THE CLIENT IS ON A CANE, WALKER OR WHEELCHAIR. YOU WILL NEED EXTRA TIME. IF THE CLOSETS ARE ORGANIZED, IT'S VERY EASY TO GET THEM DRESSED. IF THE FOOD IN THE REFRIGERATOR AND CABINETS ARE ORGANIZED AND PREPPED AHEAD OF TIME; THIS MAKES IT EASIER. MAKE A LIST OF FOOD AND DRINKS THAT NEED TO BE REPLENISHED. THIS CUTS BACK ON TRIPS TO THE STORE.

EACH CLIENT HAS A LIVING SPACE. THEY USE IT TO SIT IN THEIR FAVORITE CHAIR OR SOFA TO EAT, WATCH TELEVISION, READ OR USE THE COMPUTER. KEEP THAT AREA SANITIZED DAILY AS WELL AS THE OTHER HOUSEHOLD CHORES YOU DO DAILY LIKE: VACUUMING, COOKING, DISHWASHING, ETC. THE BATHROOM MUST BE SANITIZED DAILY AND THE HOME WILL ALWAYS SMELL FRESH.

KEEP THE CLIENT DRESSED AND FED
FIRST AND THEN CLEAN UP THE HOUSE.
BLEACH IS A VERY GOOD PRODUCT TO USE
IN ORDER TO KEEP THE HOME FRESH.

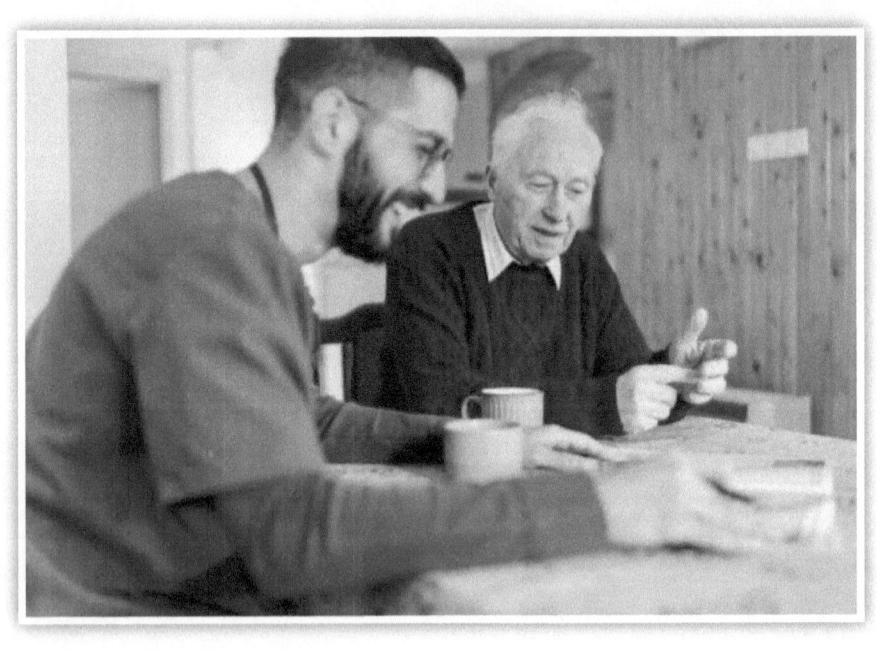

THE AVERAGE TASK OF CAREGIVERS ARE:
MEAL PREP, SANITIZING LIVING AREA,
MAKING THE BED, CLEANING LIVING ROOM,
WASHING DISHES, WIPING COUNTERTOPS,
WASHING DISHES, VACUUMING,
DUSTING, LAUNDRY, ASSISTING WITH
BATHING, ANSWERING THE TELEPHONE,
COMBING HAIR, ZIPPING BLOUSE OR
SHIRTS, APPOINTMENT REMINDERS.

CAREGIVERS NEVER HANDLE TELEPHONE CALLS, THEY ONLY ANSWER AND HAND OVER THE TELEPHONE TO THE CLIENT. IF YOU ARE ASKED TO DIAL A NUMBER, THE CAREGIVER MUST DIAL AND IMMEDIATELY HAND THE PHONE OVER TO THE CLIENT.

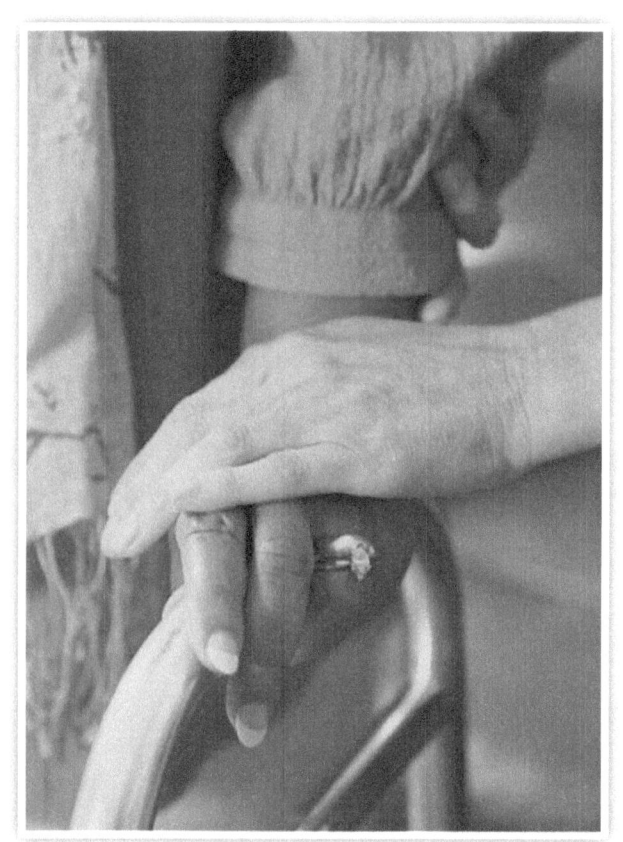

CAREGIVERS CLEAN THE REFRIGERATOR
AND STOVE ONCE A YEAR,
USUALLY CLOSE TO HOLIDAYS LIKE
THANKSGIVING AND CHRISTMAS.

YOU ARE THERE TO ONLY SERVE THE CLIENT AND NO ONE ELSE. IF YOU SEE THAT THE CLIENT'S BEHAVIOR OR CONDITION IS A THREAT TO THEIR LIFE OR YOURS, DIAL "911" AND THEN YOUR SUPERVISOR. IF THEY FALL, CALL FOR HELP AND THEN YOUR SUPERVISOR.

*

*REPORT ALL HOSPITAL VISITS TO YOUR SUPERVISOR.

*

WHEN ASSISTING THEM AND THEY USE A CANE OR WALKER, ALWAYS STAND ON THE WEAKEST SIDE IN CASE THEY BECOME WEAK AND YOU NEED TO SUPPORT THEM.

IF YOU ARE VOLUNTEERING AS A CAREGIVER
AND YOU HAVE NO SUPERVISOR –
TREAT IT AS THOUGH YOU DO.

THERE WILL BE DAYS WHERE YOU'VE
REPEATED YOURSELF TOO MANY TIMES
SO TAKE A DEEP BREATH AND USE
YOUR PATIENCE BECAUSE THE CLIENT
DOESN'T UNDERSTAND WHAT THEY
ARE DOING IN MANY CASES. DEMENTIA
CAUSES MEMORY LOSS. TELLING THEM
HOW MANY TIMES THEY'VE REPEATED
THEMSELVES DOESN'T HELP BECAUSE IN
MANY CASES, THEY WON'T BELIEVE YOU.

*

BE CAREFUL WHEN ASKED TO THROW
AWAY PAPERWORK AND ITEMS.
THE CLIENT MAY ASK YOU TO HAND
IT TO THEM A WEEK LATER.

CLIENTS GET FRUSTRATED WITH THEIR
CONDITION AND NOT BEING ABLE TO
CARE FOR THEMSELVES; SOMETIMES
A HUG CAN GO A LONG WAY.

*

AS A CAREGIVER YOU ARE VERY BUSY, SO
YOUR CLIENT MAY EVEN REMIND YOU OF
WHERE SOMETHING IS A WEEK LATER.

*

GET USE TO THE CLIENT MISPLACING
SIMPLE THINGS – AS YOU GET USE TO
BEING AROUND THEM, YOU'LL BEGIN
TO PIN-POINT EXACTLY WHERE THEY
PUT THINGS. SOMETIMES THE INK PEN
MAY BE RIGHT THERE IN THEIR HAND.

*

SOME CLIENTS CRY WITHOUT EVEN KNOWING
WHY. MOREOVER, IT COULD BE BECAUSE
SOMEONE MOVED A FAVORITE PHOTO AND
THEY WANT IT BACK WHERE IT WAS SITTING.

THE AVERAGE SENIOR SHOWERS ONCE
OR TWICE PER WEEK DUE TO WEAKNESS;
HOWEVER, FRESH WET WIPES ARE A VERY
GOOD PRODUCT TO USE FOR FRESHENING
UP BETWEEN WASHROOM VISITS.

*

YOU WILL HAVE SOME WONDERFUL DAYS
WHERE EVERYTHING IS FLOWING NICELY
AND THE CLIENT IS EVEN STRONG ENOUGH
TO LIFT THEMSELVES AND EAT WELL. IF
THERE IS NO APPETITE, NEVER FORCE IT.
IF THEY CANNOT KEEP FOOD DOWN AND
YOU FORCE THEM THEY MAY GET SICK.

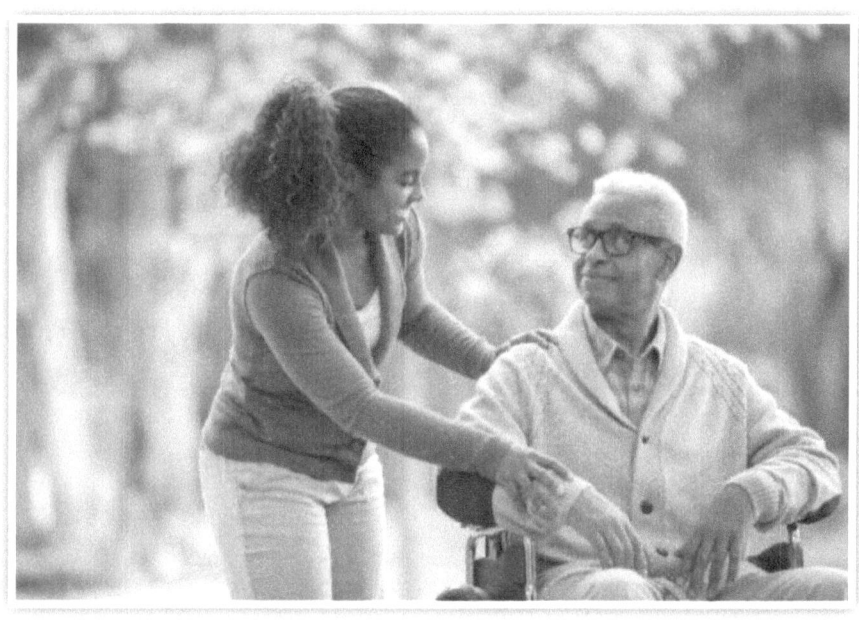

IF YOUR OWN HOME IS CLEAN BEFORE YOU ARRIVE AT YOUR CLIENT'S HOME, YOU FEEL GOOD ABOUT CLEANING SOMEONE ELSE'S HOME. THIS MAKES YOU FEEL ORGANIZED.

PRAY DAILY ABOUT YOURSELF, YOUR CLIENT,
YOUR RELATIONSHIP BETWEEN THE TWO
OF YOU AND YOU BEING AROUND THEIR
FAMILY AND FRIENDS WHEN THEY VISIT.

*

"GOD IS A REWARDER OF THOSE
WHO DILIGENTLY SEEK HIM."

WHEN YOU DO A GOOD JOB TO THE
BEST OF YOUR ABILITY, GOODNESS
WILL COME BACK TO YOU!

*

NEVER TALK FOR YOUR CLIENT DURING
DOCTOR'S VISITS. DRIVE THEM THERE
AND ONLY ASSIST THEM BY GETTING
THEM THERE AND BACK HOME.

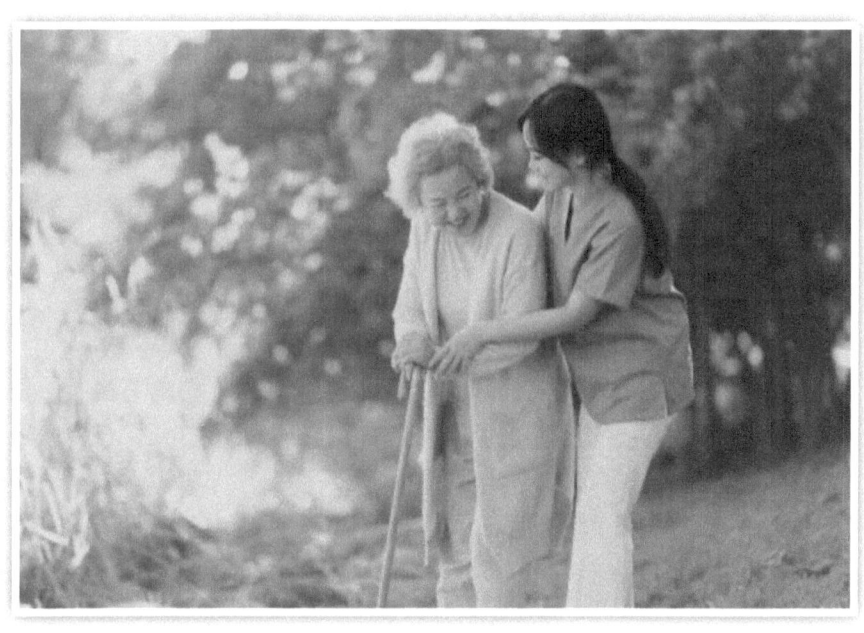

USE WISDOM REGARDING STOPPING
AT STORES OR OTHER PLACES. YOU
ARE SUPPOSED TO TRANSPORT THEM
ONLY TO IMPORTANT APPOINTMENTS
LIKE DOCTORS AND DENTISTS AND
THE STORE TO REPLENISH FOOD
OR ARTICLES OF CLOTHING.

*

IF THE CLIENT SENDS YOU TO THE STORE
WITHOUT THEM, FILL OUT THE PROPER
RECEIPTS WHICH SHOWS CASH GIVEN,
WHAT WAS SPENT AND THE AMOUNT OF
CHANGE. YOUR AGENCY GIVES YOU ALL
OF THE NECESSARY PAPERWORK.

*

AS A VOLUNTEER, MAKE A NOTE OF MONEY
GIVEN FOR TRIPS TO THE STORE AND MAKE
SURE TO GET RECEIPTS FOR PURCHASES.

REMAIN AS PROFESSIONAL AS POSSIBLE
WHILE STILL BEING COMFORTABLY ABLE
TO KEEP A GOOD RELATIONSHIP.

*

SERVE YOUR CLIENT AND NOT OTHERS.
YOU ARE HIRED TO BE A CAREGIVER TO AN
INDIVIDUAL AND NOT THEIR FAMILY AND
FRIENDS. SPEAK KINDLY TO ANY OTHERS
WHO MAY ASK YOU TO GET THEM A DRINK
OF WATER. SAY, "I AM SORRY BUT I AM
ONLY HERE TO SERVICE MY CLIENT."

SUPERVISORS PERIODICALLY SHOW
UP AT THE CLIENT'S HOME TO ACCESS
THE CAREGIVER, CLIENT AND HOME.
ALWAYS KEEP THE HOME CLEAN AND
THE CLIENT FED AND FULLY DRESSED.

*

ALWAYS DRESS APPROPRIATE AS A
CAREGIVER. SOME PREFER TO WEAR SCRUBS
AND KROCS OR GYMSHOES WITH HAIR
PINNED UP. COMFORT IS VERY IMPORTANT.

SOME CLIENTS USE VULGAR OR OFFENSIVE
LANGUAGE. ALWAYS BE PROFESSIONAL.
IF THIS BECOME UNBEARABLE
REPORT IT TO YOUR SUPERVISOR.

*

"WE WALK BY FAITH AND NOT BY SIGHT"

*

MAKE A LIST OF DAILY CHORES AND
RESPONSIBILITIES UNTIL YOU NO
LONGER NEED IT ANY LONGER.

*

EVENTUALLY YOU WILL BE HANDING
THE CLIENT THINGS BEFORE
THEY EVEN ASK FOR IT.

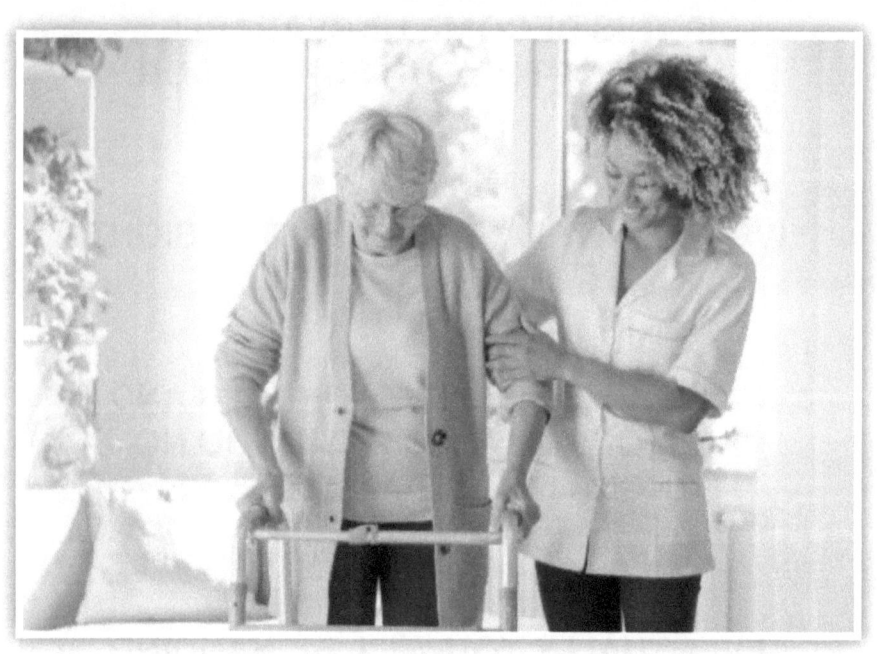

IF THE CLIENT WEAR 24/7 OXYGEN WITH A CANNULA IN THEIR NOSE, CHANGE THE CORD WEEKLY. IF THEY GET A NOSE BLEED, PUT THE CANNULA INSIDE THEIR MOUTH UNTIL YOU ARE ABLE TO STOP THE NOSE BLEED.

*

IF THE CLIENT USES THE LARGE HOME OXYGEN MACHINE, CHANGE THE 25" OR 40" CORD EVERY FEW WEEKS. ALSO, THE OXYGEN CONCENTRATOR BOTTLE HUMIDIFIER THAT'S ATTACHED TO THE MACHINE MUST BE REPLACED MONTHLY. IF IT ISN'T THEN THE MACHINE DOESN'T WORK PROPERLY AND SERVICE WILL BE CALLED MORE OFTEN THEN IT SHOULD. THE TOP TO THE CONCENTRATOR BOTTLE HUMIDIFIER MUST ALSO BE TWISTED ON THE BOTTLE EVENLY AND NOT CROOKED OR AN ALARM WILL SOUND. MANY DO NOT KNOW WHY THAT ALARM KEEPS SOUNDING; MOST OF THE TIME IT IS BECAUSE THE BOTTLE OR THE OXYGEN CORD IS LOOSE. ONLY DISTILLED WATER IS TO BE USED INSIDE OF THE BOTTLE.

NEVER TAKE PHOTOS OR VIDEOS WITH YOUR CLIENT. THAT VIOLATES THE HIPAA LAW AND IT IS GROUNDS FOR TERMINATION.

CAREGIVERS HAVE QUARTERLY
TRAINING MODULES TO ENHANCE
YOUR SKILLS. THESE VIDEOS ARE VERY
HELPFUL AND ALSO INCREASE YOUR
UNDERSTANDING ABOUT PATIENT CARE.

*

FORGIVENESS IS POWERFUL. REMEMBER
TO ALWAYS BE THE CHANGE THAT
YOU WANT TO SEE IN THIS WORLD.

THERE WILL BE DAYS WHEN THE PATIENT
ONLY NEEDS SOMEONE TO TALK TO;
THEREFORE, LISTENING IS IMPORTANT.

*

UPON RETURNING BACK HOME AT THE
END OF YOUR SHIFT; SET A CLEAR MIND
AND YOUR FOCUS ON YOURSELF.

AS LONG AS YOU ARE HEALTHY AND STRONG, YOU ARE ABLE TO TAKE CARE OF OTHERS. REMEMBER TO GET ENOUGH SLEEP, EAT HEALTHY, TAKE VITAMENS, FACIALS, HAIR, RELAXING BATHS, VACATIONS AND NEVER MISS YOUR DOCTOR'S APPOINTMENTS EITHER.

*

START YOUR DAY IN FAITH AND STAY IN FAITH!

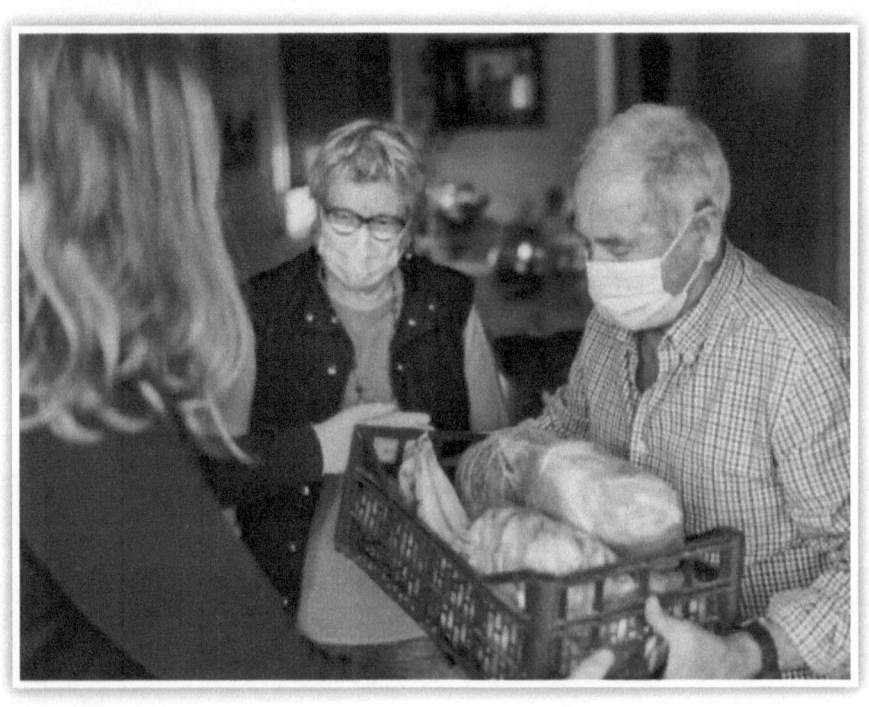

THE AVERAGE CLIENT LOSES THINGS
AND BLAME WHOMEVER IS IN THE HOME.
SUGGEST PLACES THAT YOU ALL CAN
LOOK AND BACK-TRACT WHICH USUALLY
HELP FIND THE MISSING ITEM.

AS A CAREGIVER YOU ARE NOT THE ANSWER
TO EVERY PROBLEM. DO YOUR JOB AND
MENTALLY LEAVE ROOM FOR YOURSELF.

*

ALWAYS STRIVE TO BETTER YOURSELF.
ENHANCE YOUR EDUCATION BY TAKING
CLASSES, IMPROVE YOUR HEALTH BY
JOINING AN EXERCISE CLUB. ENHANCE
YOUR BODY, MIND AND SPIRIT.

WHEN YOUR CLIENT IS TAKING A NAP, THAT IS THE BEST TIME TO STEAM OR IRON, PREPARE MEALS AND GET SOME QUIET TIME FOR YOUR SELF. TAKE A BREAK!

*

WHETHER IT IS A GOOD DAY OR A BAD DAY, DO YOUR BEST!

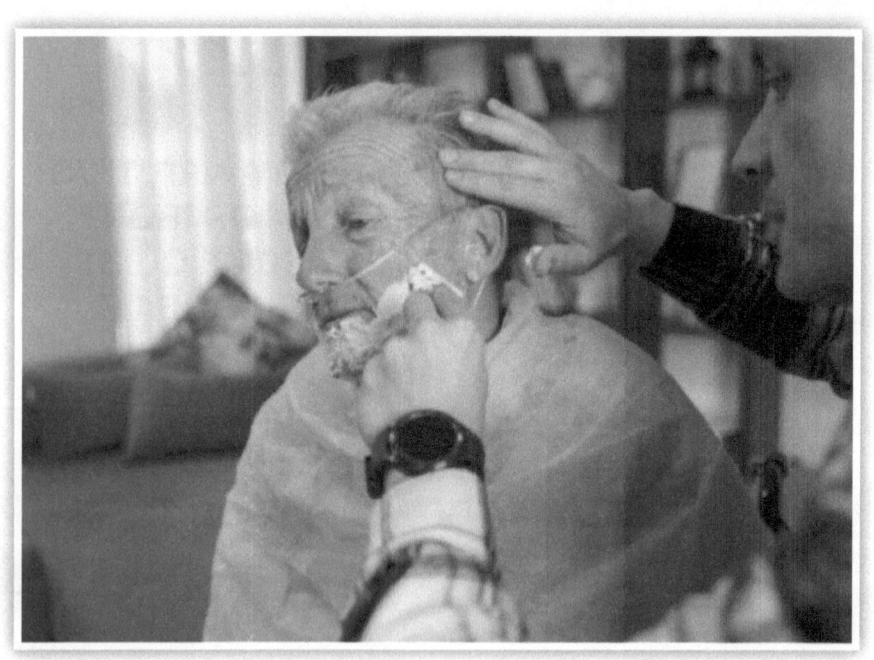

EMBRACE LAUGHTER BECAUSE ON THOSE
BAD DAYS YOU WILL FIND YOURSELF
APPRECIATING THE GOOD ONES.

*

DO ONE THING AT A TIME. SOME CLIENTS ASK
FOR 3 THINGS AT ONCE. TAKE YOUR TIME
AND DO THE MOST IMPORTANT THING FIRST.

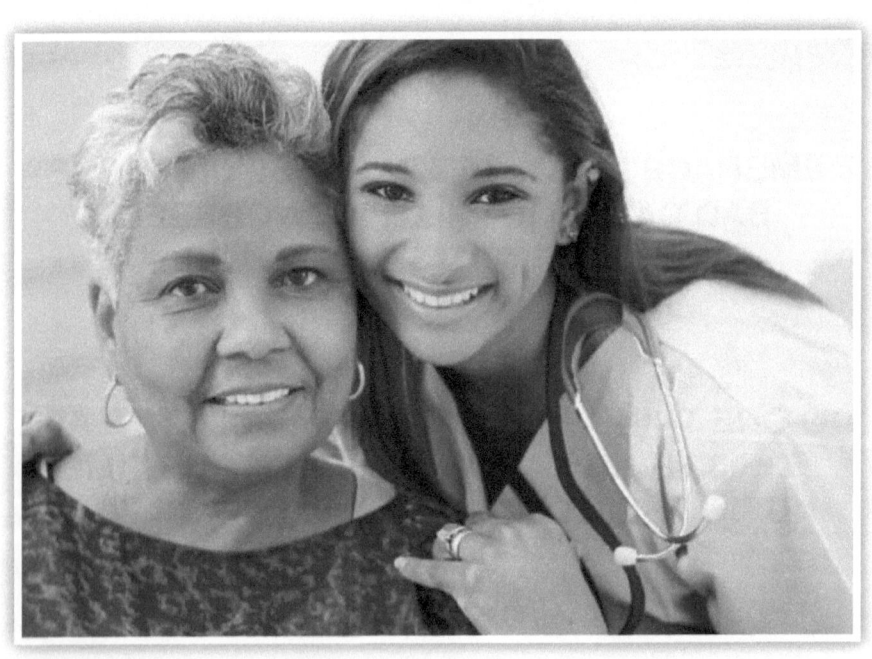

IF THEY CALL YOU AND THEN FORGET WHAT THEY CALLED YOU FOR, SIMPLY SAY, "IT'S OKAY, YOU'LL REMEMBER LATER." SOME CLIENTS CRY WHEN THEY CAN'T REMEMBER SO YOUR JOB IS TO COMFORT THEM.

EMBRACE YOUR ALONE TIME, OFF DAYS AND YOUR VACATIONS. YOU'RE AMAZING AND YOU DESERVE IT!

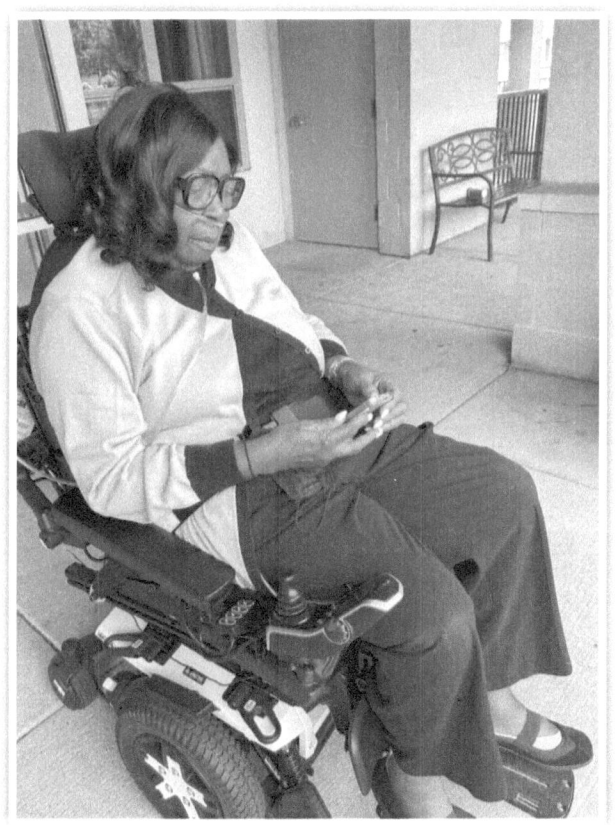

Mary's Mom

MEET A REAL MAN

Terrible things happen to unbelievers who sin; but God can transform that life. Your words can be more explosive than the atomic bomb. You can use them to destroy life or build up people. Right where you are, God is saying that He will never leave you or forsake you. That means that He is living inside of you. That is a promise from God. There are 66 books in the Holy Bible. There are a total of 1188 chapters in the bible. The center of the bible is Psalm 118. That means there are 594 chapters before Psalm 118 and 594 chapters after Psalm 118. That very center verse is Psalm 118:8, "It is better to trust in the Lord than to put confidence in man." Keep this verse in the center of your heart. The devil has been losing for a very long time. After you finish with all of this work down here, you get to have eternal life! When you have faith, you are not exempt from obstacles. Faith moves you through your problems and gets you pass troubles. You are not outside of the trouble zone, you simply have some help. You are not going to make it without Jesus. If you don't know who that is, allow me to introduce Him. He was conceived by the Holy Spirit. He led a sinless life. He took on all of our sins. He died, but then rose again. He is seated at the right hand of God the Father. Men are lost and are at the judgment of Christ. He is the One who has all Power in His hands. He is a Wonderful Counselor. He is a Mighty God. He is a Prince of Peace. He is a Savior. Oh, I know a man. He's not the cable man but He is jealous. He doesn't want us winking at no other God but Him. His name is Jesus! He is the author and finisher of our faith. You are not going to get there without Him. Do you want to be at peace in your home? Ask Him for help. Get to know Him for yourself. Include Him in everything that you do. That is how we will have a successful, peaceable life filled with relationships and love with everyone.

MEET THE AUTHOR

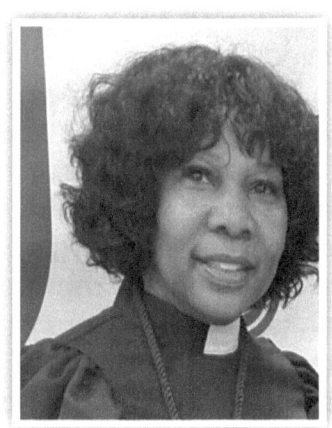

MARY BANKS is a Christian. She is also a prayer warrior. She knows that success is sharing who you are with others. Mary's mission is to tell people that God loves them and to remind them just who they are in Christ. She wants people to know that the only faith that we have is our actions and our conversation. Our desire won't mean anything to God or other people until they mean everything to us. She has taught bible classes for over 20 years and discusses the application to daily living. In her writings, she compels people to make the best out of whatever you've got. She stresses that a true Spiritual being will love and never hate anyone.

Mary accepted the Lord as her personal Savior as a young girl. She is a licensed minister who has been called to teach and evangelize about the Word of God consistently. As a part of her mandate, she traveled to hospitals on intercessory prayer missions. She also traveled state to state facilitating workshops for women and to preach the gospel. She is a notary public and made house-calls to the sick and shut-in for years. She preaches in nursing homes, prisons, helps with outreach and many other things. Mary has a bachelor's degree in management communications from DePaul University. She also has a master's degree in biblical studies. She has associates in Stenography and Legal Secretarial Science. She received her honorary Doctorate of Divinity and a second Doctorate of Philosophy. Mary retired after spending 30 years working in law enforcement as an administrator and stenographer while also serving voluntarily in various capacities in the local church. She is currently in a new career teaching at a learning center. She worked diligently in her community passing out free food, face masks and sanitizers during the covid-19 pandemic. She has volunteered as a secretary of her block club alongside her husband who is the president for many years. Mary served as a parent volunteer in the Chicago Public and Private schools. She works as a background actor for television. Her first edition of her book, "An Attitude of Expectancy" rated 8.93 by the critics and is online at Amazon. Mary enjoys writing and traveling. Her favorite exercises are walking, jogging and boxing at a sports club. She wants everyone to know that difficult situations must be examined; because it is healthy to recognize them without avoidance. In her books, she explains that some problems may be there for a long period of time in order to teach us and to see just how long it takes our hearts to become humble. She has taught her students to be the change that they want to see in this world.

www.ingramcontent.com/pod-product-compliance
Lightning Source LLC
Chambersburg PA
CBHW031501210526
45463CB00003B/1021